Fat seemed  Victoria: Tweedledum and Tweedledee; Joe "the fat boy" in *The Pickwick Papers*; even the first known report of childhood obesity in 1859. But for the short, corpulent (and extremely successful) undertaker William Banting, the overweight life was not a bundle of laughs. It was only at the age of sixty, when he was unable to even "attend to the little offices which humanity requires, without considerable pain and difficulty", that he finally stumbled upon a cure: an early incarnation of the Atkins diet. Butter, potatoes, sugar, milk—all gone, in favour of fish, meat, dry toast (and seven glasses of claret a day).

And with the diet for the body came a diet for the mind: for Lewis Carroll, an indiscriminate intake of "fatty" information was just as harmful as carbohydrates—and in today's society of ever-increasing "consumption" of food, news and even relationships, Banting and Carroll are remarkably ahead of their time.

The books in "Found on the Shelves" have been chosen to give a fascinating insight into the treasures that can be found while browsing in The London Library. Now celebrating its 175th anniversary, with over seventeen miles of shelving and more than a million books, The London Library has become an unrivalled archive of the modes, manners and thoughts of each generation which has helped to form it.

From essays on dieting in the 1860s to instructions for gentlewomen on trout-fishing, from advice on the ill health caused by the "modern" craze of bicycling to travelogues from Norway, they are as readable and relevant today as they were more than a century ago—even if contemporary dieticians might not recommend quite such a regular intake of brandy!

on
CORPULENCE

Feeding the Body
&
Feeding the Mind

The London Library

Pushkin Press

Pushkin Press
71–75 Shelton Street
London WC2H 9JQ

William Banting, *Letter on Corpulence: Addressed to the Public*. 3rd
edition. London: Harrison, 1864

Lewis Carroll, *Feeding the Mind*, with a prefatory note by William H.
Draper. London: Chatto & Windus, 1907

"A Case for Mr. Banting" by John Leech (1817–1864), published in
Punch; or, The London Charivari, May 14, 1864

"Banting in the Yeomanry" by Charles Keene (1823–1891), published
in *Punch; or, The London Charivari*, July 15, 1865

"The Working Man" by John Tenniel (1820–1914), published in *Punch;
or, The London Charivari*, May 20, 1865

First published by Pushkin Press in 2016

9 8 7 6 5 4 3 2 1

ISBN 978 1 782272 49 6

Set in Goudy Modern by Tetragon, London

Printed by CPI Group (UK) Ltd, Croydon, CR0 4YY

www.pushkinpress.com

LETTER ON CORPULENCE

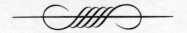

Addressed to the Public

BY WILLIAM BANTING, 1864

WILLIAM BANTING was one of the foremost undertakers of the 19th century, and was personally responsible for the funerals of both the Duke of Wellington and Prince Albert. He was a short man who suffered increasing personal distress from fatness as he aged. His dieting pamphlet, *Letter on Corpulence*, was a runaway success, and he donated all proceeds to charity. William Banting died happy and healthy in 1878, aged eighty-one.

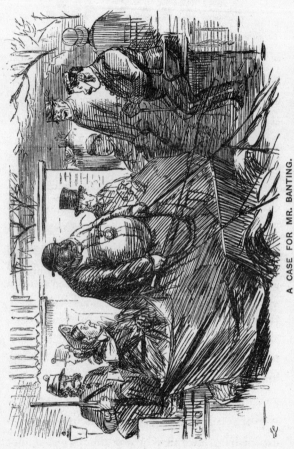

A CASE FOR MR. BANTING.

Driver (of the Herring Mould to Party inclining to embonpoint), "HOLLO, BILL! HOW MANY SACKS O' PERTATERS AND HOGSHEADS O' SUGAR 'AVE YER GOT THERE!"

Preface to the Third Edition

The second edition of this pamphlet (consisting of 1,500 copies) being exhausted, and the result being very gratifying to my mind, in the large amount of satisfaction and benefit which I am able to report from evidence of others (*beyond my most sanguine expectations*), considering the hitherto limited circulation, I have felt impelled to publish, advertise, and sell this third edition, at cost price, which I am informed must be sixpence a copy. If this small charge, however, should yield any profit, I shall devote it to the Printers' Pension Society, or some other benevolent institution; but I have no such expectation, or would very gladly reduce the charge at starting.

The first and second editions were no very serious expense to me, scarcely three pence a copy, but the circulation of them, and the correspondence involved, have cost me far more; yet, I saw no way of securing my motives from misconception except by gratuitously presenting the pamphlet to the public.

The truthful tale has, however, made its way into a large circle of sufferers with marvellous effect; and I can now believe the public will rather prefer to purchase the third edition at a reasonable charge than be under obligation to me for a gratuitous supply. I therefore humbly trust, and fully believe, that by this means the useful knowledge will be distributed twenty-fold to the benefit of suffering humanity, which, indeed, is my sole object.

KENSINGTON,
December, 1863.

This letter is respectfully dedicated to the Public simply and entirely from an earnest desire to confer a benefit on my fellow creatures.

W. B.

Corpulence

Of all the parasites that affect humanity I do not know of, nor can I imagine, any more distressing than that of Obesity, and, having just emerged from a very long probation in this affliction, I am desirous of circulating my humble knowledge and experience for the benefit of my fellow man, with an earnest hope it may lead to the same comfort and happiness I now feel under the extraordinary change,—which might almost be termed miraculous had it not been accomplished by the most simple common-sense means.

Obesity seems to me very little understood or properly appreciated by the faculty and the public generally, or the former would long ere this have hit upon the cause for so lamentable a disease, and applied effective remedies, whilst the latter would have spared their injudicious indulgence in remarks and sneers, frequently painful in society, and which, even on the strongest mind, have an unhappy tendency; but I sincerely trust this humble effort at exposition may lead to a more perfect ventilation of the subject and a better feeling for the afflicted.

It would afford me infinite pleasure and satisfaction to name the author of my redemption from the calamity, as he is the only one that I have been able to find (and my search has not been sparing) who seems thoroughly up in the question; but such publicity might be construed improperly, and I have, therefore, only to offer my personal experience as the stepping-stone to public investigation, and to proceed with my narrative of facts, earnestly hoping the reader will patiently peruse and thoughtfully consider it, with forbearance for any fault of style or diction, and for any seeming presumption in publishing it. I have felt some difficulty in deciding on the proper and best course of action. At one time I thought the Editor of the *Lancet* would kindly publish a letter from me on the subject, but further reflection led me to doubt whether an insignificant individual would be noticed without some special introduction. In the April number of the *Cornhill Magazine* I read with much interest an article on the subject— defining tolerably well the effects, but offering no tangible remedy, or even positive solution of the problem—"What is the Cause of Obesity?" I was pleased with the article as a whole, but objected to some portions, and had prepared a letter to the Editor of that Magazine offering my experience on the subject, but again it struck me that an unknown individual like myself would have but little prospect of notice; so I finally resolved to publish and circulate this Pamphlet, with no other reason, motive, or expectation than an earnest desire to help those who happen to be afflicted as I was, for that corpulence is remediable I am well convinced, and shall be delighted if I can induce others to think so. The object I have in view impels me to enter into minute particulars as well as general observations, and to revert to bygone years, in order to show that I have spared no pains nor expense to accomplish the great end of stopping and curing obesity.

I am now nearly 66 years of age, about 5 feet 5 inches in stature, and, in August last (1862), weighed 202 lbs., which I think it right to name, because the article in the *Cornhill Magazine* presumes that a certain stature and age should bear ordinarily a certain weight, and I am quite of that opinion. I now weigh 167 lbs., showing a diminution of something like 1 lb. per week since August, and having now very nearly attained the happy medium, I have perfect confidence that a few more weeks will fully accomplish the object for which I have laboured for the last thirty years, in vain, until it pleased Almighty Providence to direct me into the right and proper channel—the "tramway," so to speak—of happy, comfortable existence.

Few men have led a more active life—bodily or mentally—from a constitutional anxiety for regularity, precision, and order, during fifty years' business career, from which I have now retired, so that my corpulence and subsequent obesity was not through neglect of necessary bodily activity, nor from excessive eating, drinking, or self-indulgence of any kind, except that I partook of the simple aliments of bread, milk, butter, beer, sugar, and potatoes more freely than my aged nature required, and hence, as I believe, the generation of the parasite, detrimental to comfort if not really to health.

I will not presume to descant on the bodily structural tissues, so fully canvassed in the *Cornhill Magazine*, nor how they are supported and renovated, having no mind or power to enter into those questions, which properly belong to the wise heads of the faculty. None of my family on the side of either parent had any tendency to corpulence, and from my earliest years I had an inexpressible dread of such a calamity, so, when I was between thirty and forty years of age, finding a tendency to it creeping upon me, I consulted an eminent surgeon, now long deceased,—a kind personal friend,—who recommended increased bodily exertion before my ordinary daily labours began, and thought rowing an excellent plan. I had the command of a good, heavy, safe boat, lived near the river, and adopted it for a couple of hours in the early morning. It is true I gained muscular vigour, but with it a prodigious appetite, which I was compelled to indulge, and consequently increased in weight, until my kind old friend advised me to forsake the exercise.

He soon afterwards died, and, as the tendency to corpulence remained, I consulted other high orthodox authorities (*never any inferior adviser*), but all in vain. I have tried sea air and bathing in various localities, with much walking exercise; taken gallons of physic and liquor potasse, advisedly and abundantly; riding on horseback; the waters and climate of Leamington many times, as well as those of Cheltenham and Harrogate frequently; have lived upon sixpence a-day, so to speak, and earned it, if bodily labour may be so construed; and have spared no trouble nor expense in consultations with the best authorities in the land, giving each and all a fair time for experiment, without any permanent remedy, as the evil still gradually increased.

I am under obligations to most of those advisers for the pains and interest they took in my case; but only to one for an effectual remedy.

When a corpulent man eats, drinks, and sleeps well, has no pain to complain of, and no particular organic disease, the judgment of able men seems paralyzed,—for I have been generally informed that corpulence is one of the natural results of increasing years; indeed, one of the ablest authorities as a physician in the land told me he had gained I lb. in weight every year since he attained manhood, and was not surprised at my condition, but advised more bodily exercise—vapour baths and shampooing, in addition to the medicine given. Yet the evil still increased, and, like the parasite of barnacles on a ship, if it did not destroy the structure, it obstructed its fair, comfortable progress in the path of life.

I have been in dock, perhaps twenty times in as many years, for the reduction of this disease, and with little good effect—none lasting. Any one so afflicted is often subject to public remark, and though in conscience he may care little about it, I am confident no man labouring under obesity can be quite insensible to the sneers and remarks of the cruel and injudicious in public assemblies, public vehicles, or the ordinary street traffic; nor to the annoyance of finding no adequate space in a public assembly if he should seek amusement or need refreshment, and therefore he naturally keeps away as much as possible from places where he is likely to be made the object of the taunts and remarks of others. I am as regardless of public remark as most men, but I have felt these difficulties and therefore avoided such circum-scribed accommodation and notice, and by that means have been deprived of many advantages to health and comfort.

Although no very great size or weight, still I could not stoop to tie my shoe, so to speak, nor attend to the little offices humanity requires without considerable pain and difficulty, which only the corpulent can understand; I have been compelled to go down stairs slowly backwards, to save the jar of increased weight upon the ankle and knee joints, and been obliged to puff and blow with every slight exertion, particularly that of going up stairs. I have spared no pains to remedy this by low living (*moderation and light food* was generally prescribed, but I had no direct bill of fare to know what was really intended), and that, consequently, brought the system into a low impoverished state, without decreasing corpu-lence, caused many obnoxious boils to appear, and two rather formidable carbuncles, for which I was ably operated upon *and fed into increased obesity*.

At this juncture (about three years back) Turkish baths became the fashion, and I was advised to adopt them as a remedy. With the first few I found immense benefit in power and elasticity for walking exercise; so, believing I had found the "philosopher's stone," pursued them three times a week till I had taken fifty, then less frequently (as I began to fancy, with some reason, that so many weakened my constitution) till I had taken ninety, but never succeeded in losing more than 6 lbs. weight during the whole course, and I gave up the plan as worthless; though I have full belief in their cleansing properties, and their value in colds, rheumatism, and many other ailments.

I then fancied increasing obesity materially affected a slight umbilical rupture, if it did not cause it, and that another bodily ailment to which I had been subject was also augmented. This led me to other medical advisers, to whom I am also indebted for much kind consideration, though, unfortunately, they failed in relieving me. At last, finding my sight failing and my hearing greatly impaired, I consulted in August last an eminent aural surgeon, who made light of the case, looked into my ears, sponged them internally, and blistered the outside, without the slightest benefit, neither inquiring into any of my bodily ailments, which he probably thought unnecessary, nor affording me even time to name them.

I was not at all satisfied, but on the contrary was in a worse plight than when I went to him; however he soon after left town for his annual holiday, which proved the greatest possible blessing to me, because it compelled me to seek other assistance, and, happily, I found the right man, who unhesitatingly said he believed my ailments were caused principally by corpulence, and prescribed a certain diet,—no medicine, beyond a morning cordial as a corrective,—with immense effect and advantage both to my hearing and the decrease of my corpulency.

For the sake of argument and illustration I will presume that certain articles of ordinary diet, however beneficial in youth, are prejudicial in advanced life, like beans to a horse, whose common ordinary food is hay and corn. It may be useful food occasionally, under peculiar circumstances, but detrimental as a constancy. I will, therefore, adopt the analogy, and call such food human beans. The items from which I was

advised to abstain as much as possible were:—
Bread, butter, milk, sugar, beer, and potatoes,
which had been the main (and, I thought, inno-
cent) elements of my existence, or at all events
they had for many years been adopted freely.

These, said my excellent adviser, contain starch
and saccharine matter, tending to create fat, and
should be avoided altogether. At the first blush it
seemed to me that I had little left to live upon, but
my kind friend soon showed me there was ample,
and I was only too happy to give the plan a fair
trial, and, within a very few days, found immense
benefit from it. It may better elucidate the dietary
plan if I describe generally what I have sanction
to take, and that man must be an extraordinary
person who would desire a better table:—

> For breakfast, I take four or five ounces of
> beef, mutton, kidneys, broiled fish, bacon, or
> cold meat of any kind except pork; a large cup
> of tea (without milk or sugar), a little biscuit,
> or one ounce of dry toast.

> For dinner, Five or six ounces of any fish
> except salmon, any meat except pork, any
> vegetable except potato, one ounce of dry

toast, fruit out of a pudding, any kind of poultry or game, and two or three glasses of good claret, sherry, or Madeira—Champagne, Port and Beer forbidden.

For tea, Two or three ounces of fruit, a rusk or two, and a cup of tea without milk or sugar.

For supper, Three or four ounces of meat or fish, similar to dinner, with a glass or two of claret.

For nightcap, if required, A tumbler of grog—(gin, whisky, or brandy, without sugar)—or a glass or two of claret or sherry.

This plan leads to an excellent night's rest, with from six to eight hours' sound sleep. The dry toast or rusk may have a table spoonful of spirit to soften it, which will prove acceptable. Perhaps I did not wholly escape starchy or saccharine matter, but scrupulously avoided those beans, such as milk, sugar, beer, butter, &c., which were known to contain them.

On rising in the morning I take a table spoonful of a special corrective cordial, which may be called the Balm of life, in a wine-glass of water, a most grateful draught, as it seems to carry away all the dregs left in the stomach after digestion, but is not aperient; then I take about 5 or 6 ounces solid and 8 of liquid for breakfast; 8 ounces of solid and 8 of liquid for dinner; 3 ounces of solid and 8 of liquid for tea; 4 ounces of solid and 6 of liquid for supper, and the grog afterwards, if I please. I am not, however, strictly limited to any quantity at either meal, so that the nature of the food is rigidly adhered to.

Experience has taught me to believe that these human beans are the most insidious enemies man, with a tendency to corpulence in advanced life, can possess, though eminently friendly to youth. He may very prudently mount guard against such an enemy if he is not a fool to himself, and I fervently hope this truthful, unvarnished tale may lead him to make a trial of my plan, which I sincerely recommend to public notice,——not with any ambitious motive, but in sincere good faith to help my fellow-creatures to obtain the marvellous blessings I have found within the short period of a few months.

I do not recommend every corpulent man to rush headlong into such a change of diet, (*certainly not*), but to act advisedly and after full consultation with a physician.

My former dietary table was bread and milk for breakfast, or a pint of tea with plenty of milk and sugar, and buttered toast; meat, beer, much bread (of which I was always very fond) and pastry for dinner, the meal of tea similar to that of breakfast, and generally a fruit tart or bread and milk for supper. I had little comfort and far less sound sleep.

It certainly appears to me that my present dietary table is far superior to the former—more luxurious and liberal, independent of its blessed effect—but when it is proved to be more healthful, comparisons are simply ridiculous, and I can hardly imagine any man, even in sound health, would choose the former, even if it were not an enemy; but, when it is shown to be, as in my case, inimical both to health and comfort, I can hardly conceive there is any man who would not willingly avoid it. I can conscientiously assert I never lived so well as under the new plan of dietary, which I should have formerly thought a dangerous extravagant trespass upon health; I am very much better, bodily and mentally, and pleased to believe that I hold the reins of health and comfort in my own hands, and, though at sixty-five years of age, I cannot expect to remain free from some coming natural infirmity that all flesh is heir to, I cannot at the present time complain of one. It is simply miraculous, and I am thankful to Almighty Providence for directing me, through an extraordinary chance, to the care of a man who could work such a change in so short a time.

Oh! that the faculty would look deeper into and make themselves better acquainted with the crying evil of obesity—that dreadful tormenting parasite on health and comfort. Their fellow men might not descend into early premature graves, as I believe many do, from what is termed apoplexy, and certainly would not, during their sojourn on earth, endure so much bodily and consequently mental infirmity.

Corpulence, though giving no actual pain, as it appears to me, must naturally press with undue violence upon the bodily viscera, driving one part upon another, and stopping the free action of all. I am sure it did in my particular case, and the result of my experience is briefly as follows:—

I have not felt so well as now for the last twenty years.

Have suffered no inconvenience whatever in the probational remedy.

Am reduced many inches in bulk, and 35 lbs. in weight in thirty-eight weeks.

Come down stairs forward naturally, with perfect ease.

Go up stairs and take ordinary exercise freely, without the slightest inconvenience.

Can perform every necessary office for myself.

The umbilical rupture is greatly ameliorated, and gives me no anxiety.

My sight is restored—my hearing improved.

My other bodily ailments are ameliorated; indeed, almost past into matter of history.

I have placed a thank-offering of £50 in the hands of my kind medical adviser for distribution amongst his favourite hospitals, after gladly paying his usual fees, and still remain under overwhelming obligations for his care and attention, which I can never hope to repay. Most thankful to Almighty Providence for mercies received, and determined to press the case into public notice as a token of gratitude.

I have the pleasure to afford, in conclusion, a satisfactory confirmation of my report, in stating that a corpulent friend of mine, who, like myself, is possessed of a generally sound constitution, was labouring under frequent palpitations of the heart and sensations of fainting, was, at my instigation, induced to place himself in the hands of my medical adviser, with the same gradual beneficial results. He is at present under the same ordeal, and in eight weeks has profited even more largely than I did in that short period; he has lost the palpitations, and is becoming, so to speak, a new made man—thankful to me for advising, and grateful to the eminent counsellor to whom I referred him—and he looks forward with good hope to a perfect cure.

I am fully persuaded that hundreds, if not thousands, of our fellow men might profit equally by a similar course; but, constitutions not being all alike, a different course of treatment may be advisable for the removal of so tormenting an affliction.

My kind and valued medical adviser is not a doctor for obesity, but stands on the pinnacle of fame in the treatment of another malady, which, as he well knows, is frequently induced by the disease of which I am speaking, and I most sincerely trust most of my corpulent friends (and there are thousands of corpulent people whom I dare not so rank) may be led into my tramroad. To any such I am prepared to offer the further key of knowledge by naming the man. It might seem invidious to do so now, but I shall only be too happy, if applied to by letter in good faith, or if any doubt should exist as to the correctness of this statement.

WILLIAM BANTING, SEN.,
Late of No. 27, St. James's Street, Piccadilly,
Now of No. 4. The Terrace, Kensington.
May, 1863

Addenda

Having exhausted the first Edition (1,000 copies) of the foregoing Pamphlet; and a period of one year having elapsed since commencing the admirable course of diet which has led to such inestimably beneficial results, and, "as I expected, and desired" having quite succeeded in attaining the happy medium of weight and bulk I had so long ineffectually sought, which *appears necessary to health at my age and stature*—I feel impelled by a sense of public duty, to offer the result of my experience in a second Edition. It has been suggested that I should have sold the Pamphlet, devoting any profit to Charity as more agreeable and useful; and I had intended to adopt such a course, but on reflection feared my motives might be mistaken; I, therefore, respectfully present this (like the first Edition) to the Public gratuitously, earnestly hoping the subject may be taken up by medical men and thoroughly ventilated.

It may (and I hope will) be, as satisfactory to the public to hear, as it is for me to state, that the first Edition has been attended with very comforting results to other sufferers from Corpulence, as the remedial system therein described was to me under that terrible disease, which was my main object in publishing my convictions on the subject. It has moreover attained a success, produced flattering compliments, and an amount of attention I could hardly have imagined possible. The pleasure and satisfaction this has afforded me, is ample compensation for the trouble and expense I have incurred, and I most sincerely trust, "as I verily believe," this second Edition will be accompanied by similar satisfactory results from a more extensive circulation. If so, it will inspirit me to circulate further Editions, whilst a corpulent person exists, requiring, as I think, this system of diet, or so long as my motives cannot be mistaken, and are thankfully appreciated.

My weight is reduced 46 lbs., and as the *very gradual reductions* which I am able to show may be interesting to many, I have great pleasure in stating them, believing they serve to demonstrate further the merit of the system pursued.

My weight on 26th August, 1862, was 202 lbs.
On 7th September, it was 200 lbs., having lost 2 lbs.

27th September	"	197	"	3	"
19th October	"	193	"	4	"
9th November	"	190	"	3	"
3rd December	"	187	"	3	"
24th December	"	184	"	3	"
14th Jan., 1863	"	182	"	2	"
4th February	"	180	"	2	"
25th February	"	178	"	2	"
18th March	"	176	"	2	"
8th April	"	173	"	3	"
29th April	"	170	"	3	"
20th May	"	167	"	3	"
10th June	"	164	"	3	"
1st July	"	161	"	3	"
22nd July	"	159	"	2	"
12th August	"	157	"	2	"
26th August	"	156	"	1	"
12th September	"	156	"	0	"

TOTAL LOSS OF WEIGHT: 46 lbs.

My girth is reduced round the waist, in tailor phraseology, 12¼ inches, which extent was hardly conceivable even by my own friends, or my respected medical adviser, until I put on my former clothing, over what I now wear, which was a thoroughly convincing proof of the remarkable change. These important desiderata have been attained by the most easy and comfortable means, with but little medicine, and almost entirely by a system of diet, that formerly I should have thought dangerously generous. I am told by all who know me that my personal appearance is greatly improved, and that I seem to bear the stamp of good health; this may be a matter of opinion or friendly remark, but I can honestly assert that I feel restored in health, "bodily and mentally," appear to have more muscular power and vigour, eat and drink with a good appetite, and sleep well. All symptoms of acidity, indigestion, and heartburn (with which I was frequently tormented) have vanished. I have left off using boot hooks, and other such aids which were indispensable, but being now able to stoop with ease and freedom, are unnecessary. I have lost the feeling of *occasional faintness*, and what I think a remarkable blessing and comfort is that I have been able safely to leave off knee bandages, which I had worn *necessarily* for twenty past years, and given up a truss almost entirely; indeed I believe I might wholly discard it with safety, but am advised to wear it at least occasionally for the present.

Since publishing my Pamphlet, I have felt constrained to send a copy of it to my former medical advisers, and to ascertain their opinions on the subject. They did not dispute or question the propriety of the system, but either dared not venture its practice upon a man of my age, or thought it too great a sacrifice of personal comfort to be generally advised or adopted, and I fancy none of them appeared to feel the fact of the misery of corpulence. One eminent physician, as I before stated, assured me that increasing weight was a necessary result of advancing years; another equally eminent to whom I had been directed by a very friendly third, who had most kindly but ineffectually failed in a remedy, added to my weight in a few weeks instead of abating the evil. These facts lead me to believe the question is not sufficiently observed or even regarded.

The great charm and comfort of the system is, that its effects are palpable within a week of

trial, which creates a natural stimulus to perse-
vere for a few weeks more, when the fact becomes
established beyond question.

I only intreat all persons suffering from corpulence to make a fair trial for just one clear month, as
I am well convinced, they will afterwards pursue a
course which yields such extraordinary benefit, till
entirely and effectually relieved, and be it remem-
bered, by the sacrifice merely of simple, for the
advantage of more generous and comforting food. The
simple dietary evidently adds fuel to fire, whereas
the superior and liberal seems to extinguish it.

I am delighted to be able to assert that I have
proved the great merit and advantage of the system
by its result in several other cases, similar to my
own, and have full confidence that within the next
twelve months I shall know of many more cases
restored from the disease of corpulence, for I have
received the kindest possible letters from many
afflicted strangers and friends, as well as similar
personal observations from others whom I have
conversed with, and assurances from most of them
that they will kindly inform me the result for my
own private satisfaction. Many are practising the

diet after consultation with their own medical advisers; some few have gone to mine, and others are practising upon their own convictions of the advantages detailed in the Pamphlet, though I recommend all to act advisedly, in case their constitutions should differ. I am, however, so perfectly satisfied of the great unerring benefits of this system of diet, that I shall spare no trouble to circulate my humble experience. The amount and character of my correspondence on the subject has been strange and singular, but most satisfactory to my mind and feelings.

I am now in that happy comfortable state that I should not hesitate to indulge in any fancy in regard to diet, but if I did so should watch the consequences, and not continue any course which might add to weight or bulk and consequent discomfort.

Is not the system suggestive to artists and men of sedentary employment who cannot spare time for exercise, consequently become corpulent, and clog the little muscular action with a superabundance of fat, thus easily avoided?

Pure genuine bread may be the staff of life as it is termed. It is so, particularly in youth, but I feel certain it is more wholesome in advanced life if thoroughly toasted, as I take it. My impression is, that any starchy or saccharine matter tends to the disease of corpulence in advanced life, and whether it be swallowed in that form or generated in the stomach, that all things tending to these elements should be avoided, of course always under sound medical authority.

WILLIAM BANTING

Concluding Addenda

It is very satisfactory to me to be able to state, that I remained at the same standard of bulk and weight for several weeks after the 26th August, when I attained the happy natural medium, since which time I have varied in weight from two to three pounds, more or less. I have seldom taken the morning draught since that time, and have frequently indulged my fancy, *experimentally*, in using milk, sugar, butter, and potatoes—indeed, I may say all the forbidden articles *except beer*, in moderation, with impunity, but always as an exception, not as a rule. This deviation, however, convinces me that I hold the power of maintaining the happy medium in my own hands.

A kind friend has lately furnished me with a tabular statement in regard to weight as proportioned to stature, which, under present circumstances and the new movement, may be interesting and useful to corpulent readers:—

5 feet I should be 8 stone 8 or 120 lbs.

5	"	2	"	9	"	0	"	126	"
5	"	3	"	9	"	7	"	133	"
5	"	4	"	9	"	10	"	136	"
5	"	5	"	10	"	2	"	142	"
5	"	6	"	10	"	5	"	145	"
5	"	7	"	10	"	8	"	148	"
5	"	8	"	11	"	1	"	155	"
5	"	9	"	11	"	8	"	162	"
5	"	10	"	12	"	1	"	169	"
5	"	11	"	12	"	6	"	174	"
6	"	0	"	12	"	10	"	178	"

This tabular statement, taken from a mean average of 2,648 healthy men, was formed and arranged for an Insurance Company by the late Dr. John Hutchinson. It answered as a pretty good standard, and insurances were regulated upon it. His calculations were made upon the volume of air passing in and out of the lungs, and this was his guide as to how far the various organs of the body were in health, and the lungs in particular. It may be viewed as some sort of probable rule, yet only as an average,—some in health weighing more by many pounds than others. It must not be looked upon as infallible, but only as a sort of general reasonable guide to Nature's great and mighty work.

On a general view of the question I think it may be conceded that a frame of low stature was hardly intended to bear very heavy weight. Judging from this tabular statement I ought to be considerably lighter than I am at present: I shall not, however, covet or aim at such a result, nor, on the other hand, feel alarmed if I decrease a little more in weight and bulk.

I am certainly more sensitive to cold since I have lost the superabundant fat, but this is remediable by another garment, far more agreeable and satisfactory. Many of my friends have said, "Oh! you have done well so far, but take care you don't go too far." I fancy such a circumstance, with such a dietary, very unlikely, if not impossible; but feeling that I have now nearly attained the right standard of bulk and weight proportional to my stature and age (between 10 and 11 stone), I should not hesitate to partake of a fattening dietary occasionally, to preserve that happy standard, if necessary; indeed, I am allowed to do so by my medical adviser but I shall always observe a careful watch upon myself to discover the effect, and act accordingly, so that, if I choose to spend a day or two with Dives, so to speak, I must not forget to devote the next to Lazarus.

The remedy may be as old as the hills, as I have since been told, but its application is of very recent date; and it astonishes me that such a light should have remained so long unnoticed and hidden, as not to afford a glimmer to my anxious mind in a search for it during the last twenty years, even in directions where it might have been expected to be known. I would rather presume it is a new light, than that it was purposely hidden merely because the disease of obesity was not immediately dangerous to existence, nor thought to be worthy of serious consideration. Little do the faculty imagine the misery and bitterness to life through the parasite of corpulence or obesity.

I can now confidently say that *quantity* of diet may be safely left to the natural appetite; and that it is the *quality* only, which is essential to abate and cure corpulence. I stated the quantities of my own dietary, because it was part of a truthful report, but some correspondents have doubted whether it should be more or less in their own cases, a doubt which would be better solved by their own appetite, or medical adviser. I have heard a graphic remark by a corpulent man, which may not be inappropriately stated here, *that big houses were not formed with scanty materials*. This, however, is a poor excuse for self indulgence in improper food, or for not consulting medical authority.

The approach of corpulence is so gradual that, until it is far advanced, persons rarely become objects of attention. Many may have even congratulated themselves on their comely appearance, and have not sought advice or a remedy for what they did not consider an evil, for an evil I can say most truly it is, when in much excess, to which point it must, in my opinion arrive, unless obviated by proper means. Many have wished to know (as future readers may) the nature of the morning draught, or where it could be obtained, but believing it would have been highly imprudent on my part to have presumed that what was proper for my constitution was applicable to all indiscriminately, I could only refer them to a medical adviser for any aid beyond the dietary; assuring them, however, it was not a dram but of an alkaline character.

Some, I believe, would willingly submit to even a violent remedy, so that an immediate benefit could be produced; this is not the object of the treatment, as it cannot but be dangerous, in my humble opinion, to reduce a disease of this nature suddenly; they are probably then too prone to despair of success, and consider it as unalterably connected with their constitution. Many under this feeling doubtless return to their former habits, encouraged so to act by the ill-judged advice of friends who, I am persuaded (from the correspondence I have had on this most interesting subject) become unthinking accomplices in the destruction of those whom they regard and esteem.

The question of four meals a-day, and the night cap, has been abundantly and amusingly criticized. I ought perhaps to have stated as an excuse for such liberality of diet, that I breakfast between eight and nine o'clock, dine between one and two, take my slight tea meal between five and six, sup at nine, and only take the night cap when inclination directs. My object in naming it at all was, that, as a part of a whole system, it should be known, and to show it is not forbidden to those who are advised that they need such a luxury; nor was it injurious in my case. Some have inquired whether smoking was prohibited. It was not.

It has also been remarked that such a dietary as mine was too good and expensive for a poor man, and that I had wholly lost sight of that class; but a very poor corpulent man is not so frequently met with, inasmuch as the poor cannot afford the simple inexpensive means for creating fat; but when the tendency does exist in that class, I have no doubt it can be remedied by abstinence from the forbidden articles, and a moderate indulgence in such cheap stimulants as may be recommended by a medical adviser, whom they have ample chances of consulting gratuitously.

I have a very strong feeling that gout (another terrible parasite upon humanity) might be greatly relieved, if not cured entirely, by this proper natural dietary, and sincerely hope some person so afflicted may be induced to practice the harmless plan for three months (as I certainly would if the case were my own) to prove it; but not without advice.

My impression from the experiments I have tried on myself of late is, that saccharine matter is the great moving cause of fatty corpulence. I know that it produces in my individual case increased weight and a large amount of flatulence, and believe, that not only sugar, but all elements tending to create saccharine matter in the process of digestion, should be avoided. I apprehend it will be found in bread, butter, milk, beer, Port wine, and Champagne; I have not found starchy matter so troublesome as the saccharine, which, I think, largely increases acidity as well as fat, but, with ordinary care and observation, people will soon find what food rests easiest in the stomach, and avoid that which does not, during the probationary trial of the proposed dietary. Vegetables and ripe or stewed fruit I have found ample aperients. Failing this, medical advice should be sought.

The word "*parasite*" has been much commented upon, as inappropriate to any but a living creeping thing (of course I use the word in a figurative sense, as a burden to the flesh), but if fat is not an insidious creeping enemy, I do not know what is. I should have equally applied the word to gout, rheumatism, dropsy, and many other diseases.

Whereas hitherto the appeals to me to know the name of my medical adviser have been very numerous, I may say hundreds, which I have gladly answered, though forming no small item of the expense incurred, and whereas the very extensive circulation expected of the third edition is likely to lead to some thousands of similar applications, I feel bound, in self-defence, to state that the medical gentleman to whom I am so deeply indebted is Mr. Harvey, Soho Square, London, whom I consulted for deafness. In the first and second editions, I thought that to give his name would appear like a puff, which I know he abhors; indeed, I should prefer not to do so now, but cannot, in justice to myself, incur further probable expense (which I fancy inevitable) besides the personal trouble, for which I cannot afford time, and, therefore, feel no hesitation to refer to him as my guarantee for the truth of the pamphlet.

One material point I should be glad to impress on my corpulent readers—it is, to get accurately weighed at starting upon the fresh system, and continue to do so weekly or monthly, for the change will be so truly palpable by this course of examination, that it will arm them with perfect confidence in the merit and ultimate success of the plan. I deeply regret not having secured a photographic portrait of my original figure in 1862, to place in juxta position with one of my present form. It might have amused some, but certainly would have been very convincing to others, and astonishing to all that such an effect should have been so readily and speedily produced by the simple natural cause of exchanging a meagre for a generous dietary under proper advice.

I shall ever esteem it a great favour if persons relieved and cured, as I have been, will kindly let me know of it; the information will be truly gratifying to my mind. That the system is a great success, I have not a shadow of doubt from the numerous reports sent with thanks by strangers as well as friends from all parts of the kingdom; and I am truly thankful to have been the humble instrument of disseminating the blessing and experience I have attained through able counsel and natural causes by proper perseverance.

I have now finished my task, and trust my humble efforts may prove to be good seed well sown, that will fructify and produce a large harvest of benefit to my fellow creatures. I also hope the faculty generally may be led more extensively to ventilate this question of corpulence or obesity, so that, instead of one, two, or three able practitioners, there may be as many hundreds distributed in the various parts of the United Kingdom. In such case, I am persuaded, that those diseases, like Reverence and Golden Pippins, will be very rare.

Appendix

Since publishing the third edition of my Pamphlet, I have earnestly pressed my medical adviser to explain the reasons for so remarkable a result as I and others have experienced from the dietary system he prescribed, and I hope he may find time to do so shortly, as I believe it would be highly interesting to the Faculty and the public generally. He has promised this at his leisure.

Numerous applications having been made to me on points to which I had not alluded, in which my correspondents felt some doubt and interest, I take this opportunity of making some few corrections in my published dietary:—

I ought, "it seems," to have excepted veal, owing to its indigestible quality, as well as pork for its fattening character; also herrings and eels (owing to their oily nature), being as injurious as salmon. In respect to vegetables, not only should potatoes be prohibited, but parsnips, beetroot, turnips, and carrots. The truth is, I seldom or ever partook of these objectionable articles myself, and did not reflect that others might do so, or that they were forbidden. Green vegetables are considered very beneficial, and I believe should be adopted at all times. I am indebted to the *Cornhill Magazine* and other journals for drawing my attention to these dietetic points. I can now also state that eggs, if not hard boiled, are unexceptionable, that cheese, if sparingly used, and plain boiled rice seem harmless.

Some doubts have been expressed in regard to the vanishing point of such a descending scale, but it is a remarkable fact that the great and most palpable diminution in weight and bulk occurs within the first forty-eight hours, the descent is then more gradual. My own experience, and that of others, assures me (if medical authority be first consulted as to the complaint) that with such slight extraneous aid as medicine can afford, nature will do her duty, and only her duty: firstly, by relieving herself of immediate pressure she will be enabled to move more freely in her own beautiful way, and secondly, by pursuing the same course to work speedy amelioration and final cure. The vanishing point is only when the disease is stopped and the parasite annihilated.

It may interest my readers to know that I have now apparently attained the standard natural at my age (10 stone 10, or 150 lbs.), as my weight now varies only to the extent of 1lb., more or less, in the course of a month. According to Dr. Hutchinson's tables I ought to lose still more, but cannot do so without resorting to medicine; and, feeling in sound vigorous health, I am perfectly content to wait upon nature for any further change.

In my humble judgment the dietary is the principal point in the treatment of Corpulence, and it appears to me, moreover, that if properly regulated it becomes in a certain sense a medicine. The system seems to me to attack only the superfluous deposit of fat, and, as my medical friend informs me, purges the blood, rendering it more pure and healthy, strengthens the muscles and bodily viscera, and I feel quite convinced sweetens life, if it does not prolong it.

It is truly gratifying to me to be able now to add that many other of the most exalted members of the Faculty have honoured my movement in the question with their approbation.

I consider it a public duty further to state, that Mr. Harvey, whom I have named in the 43rd page as my kind medical adviser in the cure of Corpulence, is not Dr. John Harvey, who has published a Pamphlet on Corpulence assimilating with some of the features and the general aspect of mine, and which has been considered (as I learn from correspondents who have obtained it) the work of my medical friend. It is not.

I am glad, therefore, to repeat that my medical adviser was, and is still, Mr. William Harvey, F.R.C.S., No. 2, Soho Square, London, W.

WILLIAM BANTING.
April, 1864.

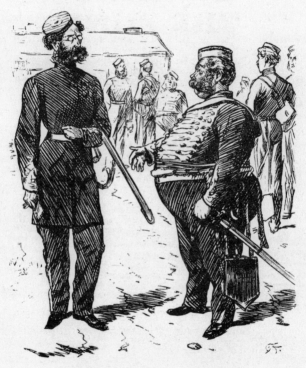

BANTING IN THE YEOMANRY.

Troop-Sergeant Major. "IT COMES TO THIS, CAPTAIN, 'A MUN E'THER HEV' A
NEW JACKET OR KNOCK OFF ONE O' MY MEALS!"

FEEDING THE MIND

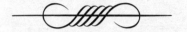

BY LEWIS CARROLL,
PUBLISHED 1907

CHARLES LUTWIDGE DODGSON, the author, mathematician and photographer, is best known as the writer of *Alice's Adventures in Wonderland* and *Through the Looking-Glass and What Alice Found There*. He was interested in, among other things, proportional representation and fair voting practices, lawn tennis and gadgets. He ate frugally, disliked tea and died in 1898.

Breakfast, dinner, tea; in extreme cases, breakfast, luncheon, dinner, tea, supper, and a glass of something hot at bedtime. What care we take about feeding the lucky body! Which of us does as much for his mind? And what causes the difference? Is the body so much the more important of the two?

By no means: but life depends on the body being fed, whereas we can continue to exist as animals (scarcely as men) though the mind be utterly starved and neglected. Therefore Nature provides that, in case of serious neglect of the body, such terrible consequences of discomfort and pain shall ensue, as will soon bring us back to a sense of our duty: and some of the functions necessary to life she does for us altogether, leaving us no choice in the matter. It would fare but ill with many of us if we were left to superintend our own digestion and circulation. "Bless me!" one would cry, "I forgot to wind up my heart this morning! To think that

it has been standing still for the last three hours!"
"I can't walk with you this afternoon," a friend
would say, "as I have no less than eleven dinners
to digest. I had to let them stand over from last
week, being so busy, and my doctor says he will not
answer for the consequences if I wait any longer!"

Well, it is, I say, for us that the consequences
of neglecting the body can be clearly seen and felt;
and it might be well for some if the mind were
equally visible and tangible—if we could take it,
say, to the doctor, and have its pulse felt.

"Why, what have you been doing with this
mind lately? How have you fed it? It looks pale,
and the pulse is very slow."

"Well, doctor, it has not had much regular food
lately. I gave it a lot of sugar-plums yesterday."

"Sugar-plums! What kind?"

"Well, they were a parcel of conundrums, sir."

"Ah, I thought so. Now just mind this: if you
go on playing tricks like that, you'll spoil all its
teeth, and get laid up with mental indigestion.
You must have nothing but the plainest reading
for the next few days. Take care now! No novels
on any account!"

*   *   *

Considering the amount of painful experience many of us have had in feeding and dosing the body, it would, I think, be quite worth our while to try and translate some of the rules into corresponding ones for the mind.

First, then, we should set ourselves to provide for our mind its *proper kind* of food. We very soon learn what will, and what will not, agree with the body, and find little difficulty in refusing a piece of the tempting pudding or pie which is associated in our memory with that terrible attack of indigestion, and whose very name irresistibly recalls rhubarb and magnesia; but it takes a great many lessons to convince us how indigestible some of our favourite lines of reading are, and again and again we make a meal of the unwholesome novel, sure to be followed by its usual train of low spirits, unwillingness to work, weariness of existence—in fact, by mental nightmare.

Then we should be careful to provide this wholesome food in *proper amount*. Mental gluttony, or over-reading, is a dangerous propensity, tending to weakness of digestive power, and in some cases to loss of appetite: we know that bread is a good and wholesome food, but who would like to try the experiment of eating two or three loaves at a sitting?

I have heard a physician telling his patient—whose complaint was merely gluttony and want of exercise—that "the earliest symptom of hyper-nutrition is a deposition of adipose tissue," and no doubt the fine long words greatly consoled the poor man under his increasing load of fat.

I wonder if there is such a thing in nature as a FAT MIND? I really think I have met with one or two: minds which could not keep up with the slowest trot in conversation; could not jump over a logical fence, to save their lives; always got stuck fast in a narrow argument; and, in short, were fit for nothing but to waddle helplessly through the world.

* * *

Then, again, though the food be wholesome and in proper amount, we know that we must not consume *too many kinds at once*. Take the thirsty a quart of beer, or a quart of cider, or even a quart of cold tea, and he will probably thank you (though not so heartily in the last case!). But what think you his feelings would be if you offered him a tray containing a little mug of beer, a little mug of cider, another of cold tea, one of hot tea, one of coffee, one of cocoa, and corresponding vessels of milk, water, brandy-and-water, and butter-milk? The sum total might be a quart, but would it be the same thing to the haymaker?

* * *

Having settled the proper kind, amount, and variety of our mental food, it remains that we should be careful to allow *proper intervals* between meal and meal, and not swallow the food hastily without mastication, so that it may be thoroughly digested; both which rules, for the body, are also applicable at once to the mind.

First, as to the intervals: these are as really necessary as they are for the body, with this difference only, that while the body requires three or four hours' rest before it is ready for another meal, the mind will in many cases do with three or four minutes. I believe that the interval required is much shorter than is generally supposed, and from personal experience, I would recommend anyone, who has to devote several hours together to one subject of thought, to try the effect of such a break, say once an hour, leaving off for five minutes only each time, but taking care to throw the mind absolutely "out of gear" for those five minutes, and to turn it entirely to other subjects. It is astonishing what an amount of impetus and elasticity the mind recovers during those short periods of rest.

And then, as to the mastication of the food, the mental process answering to this is simply *thinking over* what we read. This is a very much greater exertion of mind than the mere passive taking in the contents of our Author. So much greater an exertion is it, that, as Coleridge says, the mind often "angrily refuses" to put itself to such trouble—so much greater, that we are far too apt to neglect it altogether, and go on pouring in fresh food on the top of the undigested masses already lying there, till the unfortunate mind is fairly swamped under the flood. But the greater the exertion the more valuable, we may be sure, is the effect. One hour of steady thinking over a subject (a solitary walk is as good an opportunity for the process as any other) is worth two or three of reading only. And just consider another effect of this thorough digestion of the books we read; I mean the arranging and "ticketing," so to speak, of the subjects in our minds, so that we can read-ily refer to them when we want them. Sam Slick tells us that he has learnt several languages in his life, but somehow "couldn't keep the parcels sorted" in his mind. And many a mind that hur-ries through book after book, without waiting to digest or arrange anything, gets into that sort of condition, and the unfortunate owner finds him-self far from fit really to support the character all his friends give him.

"A thoroughly well-read man. Just you try him in any subject, now. You can't puzzle him."

You turn to the thoroughly well-read man. You ask him a question, say, in English history (he is understood to have just finished reading Macaulay). He smiles good-naturedly, tries to look as if he knew all about it, and proceeds to dive into his mind for the answer. Up comes a handful of very promising facts, but on examination they turn out to belong to the wrong century, and are pitched in again. A second haul brings up a fact much more like the real thing, but, unfortunately, along with it comes a tangle of other things—a fact in political economy, a rule in arithmetic, the ages of his brother's children, and a stanza of Gray's "Elegy," and among all these, the fact he wants has got hopelessly twisted up and entangled. Meanwhile, every one is waiting for his reply, and, as the silence is getting more and more awkward, our well-read friend has to stammer out some half-answer at last, not nearly so clear or so satisfactory as an ordinary schoolboy would have given. And all this for want of making up his knowledge into proper bundles and ticketing them.

Do you know the unfortunate victim of ill-judged mental feeding when you see him? Can you doubt him? Look at him drearily wandering round a reading-room, tasting dish after dish— we beg his pardon, book after book—keeping to none. First a mouthful of novel; but no, faugh! he has had nothing but that to eat for the last week, and is quite tired of the taste. Then a slice of science; but you know at once what the result of that will be—ah, of course, much too tough for *his* teeth. And so on through the whole weary round, which he tried (and failed in) yesterday, and will probably try and fail in to-morrow.

Mr. Oliver Wendell Holmes, in his very amusing book, "The Professor at the Breakfast Table," gives the following rule for knowing whether a human being is young or old: "The crucial experiment is this—offer a bulky bun to the suspected individual just ten minutes before dinner. If this is easily accepted and devoured, the fact of youth is established." He tells us that a human being, "if young, will eat anything at any hour of the day or night."

To ascertain the healthiness of the *mental* appetite of a human animal, place in its hands a short, well-written, but not exciting treatise on some popular subject—a mental *bun*, in fact. If it is read with eager interest and perfect attention, *and if the reader can answer questions on the subject afterwards*, the mind is in first-rate working order. If it be politely laid down again, or perhaps lounged over for a few minutes, and then, "I can't read this stupid book! Would you hand me the second volume of 'The Mysterious Murder'?" you may be equally sure that there is something wrong in the mental digestion.

If this paper has given you any useful hints on the important subject of reading, and made you see that it is one's duty no less than one's interest to "read, mark, learn, and inwardly digest" the good books that fall in your way, its purpose will be fulfilled.

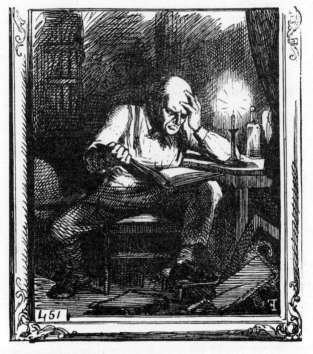

"Mental gluttony or over-reading is a dangerous propensity."

PUSHKIN PRESS—THE LONDON LIBRARY

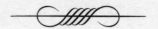

"FOUND ON THE SHELVES"

THE LONDON LIBRARY (a registered charity) is one of the UK's leading literary institutions and a favourite haunt of authors, researchers and keen readers.

Membership is open to all.

Join at www.londonlibrary.co.uk.

www.pushkinpress.com